Eating Kills
Culina Salus

First published in Great Britain in 2014 by Perseverance Works

1

Perseverance Works
presents

Eating Kills

Culina Salus

Culina Salus is a veteran of the catering industry with decades of extensive experience as a chef,chef and catering manager, event caterer ,food safety trainer working for companies such as Hilton Hotel,The BBC, Camberwell college of Arts,Tropical dream village in Malindi Kenya, Scolarest and Compass catering

Perseverance Works
presents
Eating Kills

The concise guide to eating less to save your life.
10000 kcal's of advice
No saturated fat,salt or sugar
All additives kicked out
No crap
No filler
100% original content.
Contains strong language

Introduction

This book has strong and possibly offensive language with the occasional harsh tone,you may even get outraged but taking offence should be the last thing on your mind. You are probably already dicing with your health and life with your food choices. If that is the case,then you need to consider the following:

Are you already a member of the overweight society of the UK,possibly over eating to join the super obese syndicate?

May be you have reached that point in your life where you can only see your genitals by looking in a mirror? That is not a good place to be.

May be your doctor is prescribing different types of drugs and dosages to help with your blood pressure,blood sugar and cholesterol levels? ailments brought on by your lifestyle choices. You have eaten yourself into becoming a drug addict.

May be you have been refused surgery or a procedure,due to your weight or blood pressure levels.

May be you are so unhealthy and unfit, a three year old could easily outrun you?

May be you have left the world of fitted clothes behind and only deal in baggy tracksuits now?

May be you do not see anything wrong in eating a 1500 kcal fast food meal in one sitting. On a regular basis.

May be you are on first name terms with the owner of the big and mighty clothing superstore.

May be you cannot bear to look at your naked body in the mirror.

Offensive language? least of your problems right now, in this age,where people are getting seriously ill and dying from simply eating much,tone of language is not an issue.

Everything you read from this point on is just personal opinion and observation, if you want qualified medical advice? go see your doctor,not that you'll take their advice ,otherwise you wouldn't need to see them, would you now?

Saving money on your weekly food shop is not just about being prudent with your purchasing power but it is really about changing your mindset. As we need to eat to live, it is prudent to learn to buy the right stuff.

Its about the power of making a decision and sticking to it,in the face of all temptation. At one moment in time,you have an epiphany and resolve to become a vegetarian and 10 years later,you are still meat free,or you see a picture of yourself in a holiday snap,and you cannot recognise the person bursting out of the swimming outfit,if you are lucky a neon sign goes off in your head,flashing enough is enough and you start taking action to resolve your runaway eating habit. That is the power of making a life changing decision;to decide to go against the grain for the betterment of your life.

And it is just that,an eating habit,not a taste and enjoy the food habit,not an eat to sustain your life habit but just an eating habit,moving your mouth non stop.

A very bad habit;mouth moving as an activity.

One of the best meal combinations was meat,potatoes and two veg, it was a well balanced meal,a combination of protein,carbohydrates and vegetables,the closest thing we had to the "eat well" or "diet plate". Now it is more likely that your main meal is just slices of pizza,takeaways centred around rice, southern fried chicken and chips or a ready meal,all carbs,a minuscule portion of protein with no vegetables in sight. With the popularity of chilled and frozen ready meals,it means that content and portion size is out of our control. May be you are one of the few that add salad or vegetables to your chilled,frozen and takeaway meals?

The previous generation did not eat as well as we do,their food choices were not as wide ranging and possibly unlimited as it is today, but they were much more active,
children walked to school,adults walked everywhere,snacking between meals was rare,they cooked their own meals from scratch and consequently were not as obese as we are now and lived much longer than this increasingly overweight generation ever will.

On the other hand, they never had to face the onslaught of food advertising that we do today. Our forebears never had to face the temptation of a hamburger sandwich could be ready to eat, from chilled to ready in 60 seconds. There is no time lag between your desire and fulfilment, no time to wonder, am I really hungry? Can't I wait until dinner? is this good for me?, do I really need to eat this now? how long will it take to burn off all the calories? God knows that it is easier to consume a calorie than to burn one.

This book is about reducing your food shopping budget and making smart buying decisions,in order to live a long healthy life and avoiding the life sucking,health reducing,illness inducing monstrosities disguised as food.

This is not one of those live on £1 a day nonsensical publicity stunts,that celebrities, politicians do for a very short period of time, to prove some kind of irrelevant point,anybody can survive on £1 a day for 5 days,if you know on the sixth day,you can go back to your real life and comfortably afford a steak dinner washed down with the finest red you can afford.

People taking part in such silly stunts, know there is a light at the end of the tunnel, but in certain parts of the world where people have to exist on small amounts of food and money, they have no idea where their next meal is coming from, they aren't even sure if they will be able to afford one.
These unfortunate millions live with an absence of hope, there is no light at the end of the tunnel, and if there is one, it is likely to be another calamity rushing their way. They do not have a hope of a better tomorrow, a prosperous existence or living a better life. Most of the time, they hope for some miracle from a deity, to improve their lot, whilst producing cheap foods for the atheists in the west, who are getting sick and dying from living the good life. The "good life" their deity is yet to bestow upon them.

A while back in a particular African country, there was a popular joke during a very tough period of austerity measures, on how many meals you could afford in a day. 0 meant no meals and 1 was a meal, so if you were 100, meant you could afford breakfast but nothing for lunch and dinner. 001 was dinner only and 111, well you were living large, able to afford all 3 meals daily.

But I digress, back to the futility of silly stunts, who the hell wants to endure a horrible commute to work, where you dislike your boss, despise your colleagues and hate the customers you have to deal with, then on the journey back home, on the tightly packed train, you are stuck close to an armpit of a sweaty smelly individual, who is averse to the idea of the daily shower. You finally get home and then you sit down to a £1 meal to prove your solidarity with the worlds poor.

W T F !, Hell no !.

You want to reward yourself with the best food you can afford and not indulge in some spurious exercise to identify and feel the pain of the poor and starving of the world. That is the job of various charities based in the western world, who make a good living doing such things.

Lets get to it.

1 You work hard for your money, you have to take a lot of crap at work ,just to get paid. So when it comes to food shopping, you have the god given right to decide what goes into the shopping trolley, not your whingeing, demanding, truculent and moaning kids.
Just imagine how much money, you would save, if you had enough backbone, not to submit to their harassment, embarrassing
behaviour, sulking, screaming, tantrums,
nagging, badgering or tricks.
You should not become a slave to your child's demands, you should choose what is eaten in your house. NEVER let your child send you on a guilt trip, for as long as they are well fed, clothed, healthy, loved and cared for, that's the real stuff that matters, everything else is just gravy. If the little bugger refuses the meal before them, they should stay hungry until the next meal time. There are millions of children around the world that survive on much less. Besides your

precious is probably already overweight in any case,so missing a meal may be a good thing.

You have the right and power to say no to your child's demands and tantrums,there is no need to feel guilty or anxious (you've already fed the little fuckers so well that they have plenty of energy to annoy you),no is fucking no. Saying no will never harm a child but saying yes after being brow beaten is down right irresponsible(or even weak).Saying no does not mean that you are a bad parent.
No, is probably the greatest word in the English language,no in this context means so much, it is shorthand for saying so little but meaning so much more;
No! (you can't have it)
No! (I can't afford it)
No! (I'm in a bad mood,so you ain't getting nothing)
No! (You forced me to buy some last week,I'm not giving in this time)
No! (I've got other problems to worry about,buying you chocolate is not on my to do list)
No! (leave me alone)
No! (I'm in the mood for a fight)
No!(just shut up)
No! (Fuck off)
No! (You have been pissing me off all day)
No!(I have had a shitty day at work,leave me in peace)
No!(I did not get any last night,why should you get what you want?)
No! (Its not good for you)
No! (I hate your father)
No! (You look like your nagging mother)
No! (I hate coming here)
No! (I'm depressed,I might just end up eating it myself and putting on weight).
No! (these prices are a rip off)
No!(We have some at home)
No! (I'm not in the mood to endure supermarket hell)
No! (Your food choices are so wrong)
No!(I'm not in the mood to deal with your shit now)
No!(go away,the film has just got to the good part)
No! (No means no)

"No" is a great word,that needs to be used so much more.

The enforcement officers from the department against bad parents will not come and drag you out of bed in the early hours of the morning to interrogate you about what you did or did not feed your child,but if you are giving your child, Haribo and Red bull for breakfast,a packet of crisps and Mars bar for lunch and a cheap value pizza for dinner,washed down with a value/essentials/economy fizzy drink,so cheap that the manufacturers could not be bothered to put sugar in it,then you should be locked up.

Just think how much money would stay in your bank account,if you did not buy stuff,you the hard working earner did not want or need. Stop buying all those sugary drinks,let your children get used to drinking water-there's a money saver right there. Another bonus point is that water cannot make them hyperactive and get on your nerves.

The public meltdown will probably happen,with your ray of sunshine screaming their little heads off,with you furious and feeling embarrassed at the same time,unable to clout the little fucker around the head because of the nosey onlookers.

Well, fuck the onlookers, they should mind their own damn business,you stick to the primary rule,NEVER GIVE IN,eventually your child will know that you are not to be fucked with and cannot be blackmailed to give in.
Never give in,never give ground,stand firm, you are the responsible parent and not their play mate.

Your children, know who the boss kid is on the school playground,the bully during lunch time,and they know how to stay on the right side of this nut case. You better get some balls and be the boss in your own house. So next time you go shopping,with them,as soon as they kick off,look them in the eye,give them the thousand yard stare and tell them to drop dead.

We do not negotiate with terrorists.

Or just do all your shopping online ,no fuss,no hassle,no trolley wars,no swivel eyed loons, and thank God,no screaming kids.

2 Send a man with a shopping list,take advantage of the popular myth,that men cannot multi task,that they tend to have one track minds. When a man wants sex you know,he ain't stopping till he gets some. Now just get him to bring that same focus and determination to food shopping.
He will only purchase what's on the shopping list,nothing more,nothing less. He will not be distracted by bogofs,new products,discounts or any other tempting crap,heck he will not even choose an alternative,if a particular item on the list is out of stock.
Men shop,like they have sex,a quick in and out,no time wasted,straight to the point.
Get a man to shop and see the savings start to pile up.

3 In the UK we spend over £5.5billion on takeaway meals such as Indian,pizza,burgers ,fried chicken shops and Chinese(who incidentally do not eat Chinese take away type foods) or KFC which tend to staffed by slim people from the Asian subcontinent (looking at their size,they obviously do not eat what they sell,what should that tell you?).

Takeaway meals may be tasty(saltly?) and filling but they are often relatively expensive,poor value for money,fatty,oily and saltly,often containing far more calories than you need in one meal. Also the anticipation of the meal often exceeds the pleasure of the meal.
Pop in to KFC,order a Supercharger burger(674K),large fries(450K),large coleslaw(305k) and a milky bar krushems(430K) that is a straight 1859 kcal's in one sitting,1859kcals out of a daily recommended total of 2000kcals,1859

kcal's from just one meal out of a possible three. What are you going to eat for the rest of the day? a stick of celery?

Why do the meals have so many calories? what the fuck for?,its not as if you are going on a trek to the north pole,and need to build up a layer of fat by consuming 5000 calories a day. No, you are going back to sit at your desk,drive home and have another calorie jacked dinner,then spend the rest of evening on the couch in front of the TV still snacking, Is it is any wonder that people are eating themselves to death? its so fucking easy to do.

Takeaways and fast food might be time savers,another debatable point but they sure as hell not good for you,if eaten on a regular basis.
Save your money,avoid takeaways,you would have to empty the contents of your fridge to cook a 1859 calorie meal yourself.

Look at yourself in the mirror,do you need to spend money on another high calorie fast food meal? Are your ribs sticking out? Do you look malnourished? does your body look like it is deprived of nutrition? Have you been starved?

4 lets not deceive ourselves,food is a drug,eating is addictive, some people get more pleasure from eating than having sex(shame). Hell you may not even be able to get a good shag, then you are sure going to get pleasure from that pizza topped with everything ,a scrumptious cupcake or belly busting Friday night takeaway.
Probably for some people, thinking about food is as exciting as getting turned on. Ready meals and snacks laced with salt,saturated fat are really tasty and moreish,once you throw in that bad boy sugar,then all hope is lost.
Sugar is the most addictive substance in the world, bar none, there are more sugar addicts in the world than any other substance. Scientists say that sugar stimulates the parts of the brain that cocaine does as well. Once you come to accept this,then realising that supermarkets are more dangerous than a crack dealers den, is a step in the right direction.
Buying food with care is half the job,if you don't buy the crap,you won't have to eat it and later see the stuff manifest on your waist line,clog up your arteries and make you a frequent user of the NHS. All those eye catching supermarket displays only have one purpose; to get you to increase your spending,unfortunately this leads to a bigger waistline.
We have to eat to live,but we must never forget that food,especially salty,sugary and fatty junk food is moreish and more addictive than crack cocaine,alcohol and tobacco put together.
Look around you,there are more overweight and obese people getting on high calorie junk food,than smoking,alcoholic crack heads.
The most frightening aspect is that food is still not seen as dangerous or life destroying as drugs,tobacco or alcohol. But as more people are now dying of diet related illnesses than any other factor,eating is now the most dangerous activity on the planet,bar none. Maybe,we should stick a "consume with care" label on the usual suspects.

5 Stop feeding your mindless eating habit. How is it,that when you are eating meals you have cooked from scratch, you enjoy the whole meal, savouring

every mouthful until the last bit is polished off,you have a similar experience when you go to a fine dining restaurant. You savour the textures,balance of herbs,spices,taste and quality of the food,not the quantity heaped on your plate.

There is no way that the first mouthful tastes as good as the last one at the all you can eat buffet. If you focus on the quality and not the quantity of what you eat,it will do your health a world of good.

In the case of junk food,after the first couple of bites,your taste buds switch off,your mind wanders away from the pleasure sensation,you just continuously stuff your mouth until the plate or packet is empty.

Consequently with your mind disengaged and engrossed by the television, you eat a lot more than you should have. So when you are buying big bags of crisps(made for sharing but you can easily finish the packet yourself),boxes of cakes,microwavable meals and snacks etc., it is only to feed this mindless eating habit,the habit of not enjoying the food but just stuffing your face.

A habit of keeping your mouth chewing and ignoring the feeling that you are satisfied.

6 This one is quite simple,build up your shopping list over the week,when you hit the supermarket,do not deviate from it for any reason.

Supermarket promotions have been deliberately set up to make you discard your carefully compiled list,at the first sight of an offer. After all they are the showroom for food manufacturers.

Offers only exist to make you increase your weekly spending,gimmicks such as spend £20,get £2 off,3 for the price of 2,buy one get one free or spend £40 and get 5p off a litre of petrol,are subtle ways to make you spend more.

So make your shopping list at at home and do not depart from it.... better still shop online and never enter a supermarket again. In 2013, with the current state of internet shopping, with almost EVERYTHING now sold online,you probably never need to enter a shop to buy anything again. Except to get your fast food fix, KFC,McDonald's don't do home delivery, unlike other fast foods,their creations don't travel well or last long. I wonder why.

7 Be on your guard. Supermarkets look nice,are bright,convenient and comfortable,they are really enemy territory,they are not there for your benefit. They provide all the things you need,but work hard at getting you to spend on your wants.

Their aim is to get you to spend more than you want to,can afford to or need to and sometimes less than you should. Think alcohol prices.

They are the high street in one large grey shed,with multiple mini shops covering; electronics ,mobile phones books,toys,entertainment,clothes,cosmetics,babies,car accessories, opticians,bakery,off licence,pharmacy,dry cleaner,post office, financial products,restaurants and of course food. Lets not forget the attached petrol station.

In short the high street has closed down, half of the shops have moved into a large grey shed,whilst the other half has moved online.

Supermarkets providing convenience at it best,everything you require in one place with free unrestricted parking.

Learn to navigate the supermarket assault course without spending more than you planned or I repeat,shop online and spend the time saved going on a 10000 step walk.

8 Go stand in front of a mirror. Take off your clothes. Look at yourself,really take a good look at yourself from head to toe,study all those curves,bulges,droops,stretches,can you afford to miss a meal?.Be honest with yourself. If the most likely answer is yes,then miss a meal,voilà,you have saved money.
Out of 21 meals a week,you can afford to miss a meal here and there. It will do your wallet and health a world of good, it will also strengthen your self discipline and increase self confidence.
It will make the impossible,seem possible,really? of course it will,after all you never thought you could survive missing a meal.

9 Cook your own damn food!,it is cheaper and better nutritionally than any takeaway,chilled or frozen meal. You are sure not going to add any sugar to any tomato sauce or curry that you cook from scratch at home, unlike the ready made versions. It is highly unlikely to contain as much fat or calories .
Leftovers from your cooking experiments can be put in kids lunch boxes or taken to work instead of buying that super expensive cold sandwich or over priced canteen lunch.
There will not be any requirement to read the label for any mysterious contents,as you have hand picked every ingredient yourself. You will certainly never use stuff that has never,ever been used in a domestic kitchen.
Majority of us given a choice,prefer "handmade" items, "handmade" is a sign of a premium product,made by a human being with care and attention using the best products. It is a cut above everything else,different and better. So why don't do we apply that philosophy to the food we eat,instead of chomping down every thing spewed out of a factory. The sustenance that keeps us alive and healthy,we have relegated to the realm of factories,cheapest ingredients and poorly paid workers.
Besides who really knows, what is in ready made meals? the manufacturers sure as hell don't. They hope the cheapest supplier in their food chain is honest.
The government is too spineless to legislate that the ingredients list matches the contents, and food manufacturers and retailers are experts at making apologies after the fact. They spend more time and resources putting out apologies than making sure that their methods and products are kosher.

10 Get some knife skills,buy a good knife,get a steel to keep it sharpened. You can Google it,YouTube it or book it, to skill up on how to use a knife in the kitchen. With these skills,you can chop your vegetables,peel your potatoes,cut up a whole chicken,it cheaper than precut packs.
A stir-fry for example,is all about knife skills.

11 Get some maths skills,use a calculator to check the supermarket prices,what prices? you may ask,they are clearly displayed. The advertised price is irrelevant,what is the price per kilo,gram or litre? Have you noticed that supermarkets have tried to throw you off track, by listing similar products side by side but changing the pricing details,one product is listed price per kilo,but the one next to it is listed price per 100 grams. This slight blurring of price and contents,is designed to confuse up your price comparison habits. Get your brain in gear,download an app,get smart,price per size can be applied to buying cereals,vegetables,meat,fish,in fact anything that has measurable dimensions. Can't be bothered take a calculator shopping,use the one on your smart phone dummy.

12 BOGOF aka buy one get one free,buy 3 for the price of 2,buy 1 get 2 free,buy 1 get 1 half price,get 30%,50% or even 75% more. All of these bargains,will only end up blowing you up (size wise) and drain your wallet in the process. Supermarkets do not think you are stupid but they count on your apathy,laziness and greed not to look twice at their deals and to take all offers at face value. So watch out, supermarket offers can blow you up and clean you out.
Caveat Emptor will always apply.

13 Supermarkets lead,people follow. They claim that it is the other way,that their job is satisfying customer demand,nope they create habits,desires and trends with marketing,using social media and advertising. I wonder which set of customers asked for Philadelphia cream cheese with chocolate, or 1270kcal KFC mighty bucket for 1.
Almost every company has a twitter or facebook account,in order to connect to the right audience and turn them into customers.
They lead, you follow,through marketing,public relations,social media and advertising,they create trends,would you have even thought a Christmas pudding with an whole orange stuck inside was desirable unless Waitrose had determined that it was?
Manuka honey, Acai berries,green tea,red bush tea,3 bird roast, the latest so called "super foods"how did you come to hear about these things?

Question;when was the last time,you had an independent,original thought on how to spend your money?

14 Biggest is not best when it comes to food,it just means an extra large portion of the stuff that is draining your pocket and slowly ruining your health. With food,value means more,but not necessarily better."Value" is really more added fat,cheap fillers,mock products,excess salt and sugar in short, fatcrap. These larger portions as to be expected,contain more calories.

A couple of years ago,there was a short lived furore about super sized portions of foods,where one portion of food,served to one person was enough to fully satisfy two. As always, it was the usual suspects;factory manufactured fast food,no one is super sizing a healthy salad or freshly grown produce.

As a result,the food industry focused more on multi buys,multi buy is super sizing by any other name and it always tends to be mainly the usual bad boys: junk food,snacks,sweets,crisps,soft drinks and beer.

Meal deals offered by KFC, Mcdonalds and other fast food chains are also super size offerings but disguised as "meals" ,Supercharger meal (1290kcal),Gladiator box meal (1340 kcal), Wicked zinger meal(1075),Big daddy meal (1495kcal)Big Mac meal (1160 kcal) are offerings with more calories than anybody requires in a meal at one sitting. All accompanied with mini buckets of sweet soft drinks.

This relatively cheap, energy dense food and drink is taking its toll on our health and well being, due to our mainly sedentary lifestyles,the government needs to introduce legislation than prevents any food seller from selling calorie jacked food,in that instance, McDonald's will be legally prevented from selling any burger than had more than 300kcal or a meal combination that offered more than 800 calories,a third of the daily calorie requirement. The same way some painkillers are regulated for public safety.

If people wanted to overdose on calories,they would have to buy more than one meal, go to more than one restaurant to do it,as it would not be offered in one meal.

The following signs would be displayed in every restaurant:

"For the health of our customers,we will not sell any single item or a combination of items that contain more than 800kcal per customer at one time.

15 The world is not ending. The Apocalypse is not coming,The Mayans were wrong. The end is not nigh. Armageddon ain't happening. A famine is not coming(at least not to your part of the world).

so

STOP EATING SO MUCH.

The food supply is not running out,food scientists will create more,if required. You have no reason apart from greed to consume so many calories and store up all that excess fat,it is not required to keep you warm during the winter months,suitable clothing and central heating will do that.

There are no famines in the affluent parts of the world,they can just import whatever they need,they can even afford to bin it,if it does not look sexy enough.

The victims of famines are the poor,in strife torn areas or whose environment has turned against them and they cannot ameliorate the situation as they cannot afford to buy products from the production line of the mad scientist.

On the other hand,here in the west,bursting with a wide range of goodies,the shelves are full,the supermarkets are opened 24 hours a day,full of shoppers buying and eating as if their lives depended on it.

There are food outlets EVERYWHERE,you are literally tripping over them. a burger shop is next to a chicken shop,next to a sandwich bar,then a coffee

shop,next to a supermarket express shop,next to a bakers,next to a 99p store which is not too far from the mega supermarket which is open 24 hours.
This easy access,over consumption and over spending means we are eating ourselves to death,wasting food and enormous amounts of money whilst doing it. On the other side of the world,the poor are watching,astonished that whilst they are dying from hunger and malnutrition,the people from across the water are dying from eating too much.

16 In the pursuit of greater market share,the food industry does not have its customers best interests at heart,in order to maximise the returns to their shareholders, their aim is getting us to eat whatever Frankenstein creation,they can convince us to eat. If they could successfully persuade us that sprinkling dead dried red ants on our food, had health benefits,they would.
Never forget that these are the same jokers that fed herbivore cattle, meat and bone meal made from the remains of dead cattle. For thousands of years,cattle had fed on grass but along comes some cost cutter,who turns nature on its head,in search of greater profit margins.

The usual suspects, have packed food with additives,artificial colours,added hydrogenated fats to almost everything,added cochineal extract(pulverised insects) to foods,beverages and sold us horse meat as beef,and poured high fructose corn syrup into an increasing number of foods such as soft drinks, sauces,salad dressings,soups,cakes pastries,ice cream,yoghurt and breakfast cereals. Some of the above have only been removed as they were no longer profitable,cheaper alternatives had been created or to avoid bad publicity and even create good publicity. "we have done away with saturated fats" or " our beef is sourced from the UK" are instances that come to mind.

The food industry is feeding us to death,with you and I, picking up the bill for our poor health,a result of non stop eating of fatcrap foods.
Once they have wiped us out with strokes,heart attacks,cancer,diabetes and obesity,
in order to survive and protect their bottom line,they will move onto our children and new emerging markets. The food companies are salivating at thought of 1.3 billion Chinese drinking sugary soft drinks instead of tea or 1.2 billion Indians eating pizza instead of chapati's.
Why isn't the government fighting an effective battle on our behalf ? as the food industry bombards us with fat crap food products. Rare is the child or adult who does not have a sweet tooth, has anybody ever wasted a chocolate cake ? has a packet of chocolate digestives ever sat at the back of the cupboard lonely and unwanted like a jar of Marmite?

Well, the government is not for the people but for the food industry as your elected official needs to earn a well paid living after the political life is over. Being a life long politician and never having done any other job,they are essentially unemployable,unless their friends in business and industry, come to their rescue.

A government elected by the people should be more committed to protecting the health of the public than protecting the profits of their friends in the food industry,for many elected officials,the attraction of a well paid directorship is hard to ignore,so why make enemies of the industry that will put large amounts of money in your pocket after you have been thrown out of office.

After all have you ever heard of an former member of parliament now working as a shop manager?

Interlude; what the food industry thinks of you:

They will provide a small range of healthy options,knowing that you will always be attracted to the tasty filling junk,so we have hamburgers,hot spicy chicken wings at 99p, but cucumber sold at £1. Junk food is cheap and more convenient than
healthy options.(tastier also)

If alcohol or soft drinks are cheaper than water,you will buy it,just think about the price of multi pack beer per litre vs 1 litre bottle of water.
If you buy it,you will eat it.(well most of it,as we waste 7.2 million tonnes of food a year)
if a celebrity tweets about it,you will buy it.
If it is discounted,you will buy it.
If a celebrity chef uses an ingredient in a popular recipe,you will clear the shelves.
If it is super sized,you will buy it.
If it says "new" or "improved" you will buy it.
If it is a bogof offer,you will buy it.
If it is marked down,you will buy it

The food industry has you by the short and curlies,so stop being a mugu(google it),do not fall for the obvious tricks.

End of interlude.

17 The more promises a product makes,the higher,the price but it does not necessarily mean that product is better is better for you. Some products just have an image problem,like burgers, whilst some have great P R. for example smoothies have more calories than coke,a yoghurt crunch smoothie has more calories than a donut ,even some so called healthy options are guilty of this for example McDonald's deli choices' Spicy Veggie sandwich has more calories at 520kcal than the popular bad boy,the Big Mac at 490kcal.

18 Organic has a great image,it suitably costs more but is it actually better for you? are you spending more money than you should, to get fat. Maybe organic is just a salve to your conscience,it is definitely a fashionable,dinner party conversation topic,it makes you feel better,one up on the great unwashed,who just buy all the stuff grown with horrible fertilisers. Ask yourself,does organic produce actually taste better? does it taste like the real thing? do you even know what the real thing tastes like? have you ever eaten

the real thing? Like fruit grown without fertilisers and allowed to ripen on the tree,under the sun and not in a temperature controlled warehouse? is it money well spent?,is it really healthy?,who really benefits from the organic label? Are they just charging more for food grown in bullshit?

19 The food manufacturers and retailers hate regulation mainly because if properly drafted, it can be very effective. Mayor Bloomberg of New York tried to introduce legislation to ban the sale of super-sized sugary sodas. As influential and savvy as he is ,The mayor was defeated by the well funded soft drinks lobby. Over the cold dead body of the food and drink industry will they allow, anyone to introduce legislation that was not in their interests. As always they put forward an eloquent,mild mannered spokesperson to defend their products and actions. All culpability for the obesity epidemic is denied,with claims that it is unfair,incorrect,unjust to blame the spread of diet related diseases just on their products.(a half truth,they made it,we brought it)

Politicians also hate regulation, for them it just creates enemies. The majority of politicians are not like the rest of us,amongst their many detestable qualities,is they tend to have close friendships with big business. They are happy to be lobbied over a very expensive meal. They accept gifts,directorships,memberships,consultancies and jobs, all legal and above board of course.
Your career politician needs to earn a living after the political life is over,so cultivating friendships with business leaders is essential. Whilst in office,they will rescue undeserving banks,privatise industries,introduce ineffective light touch regulation, offer subsidies or even kick issues into the long grass.

The tobacco industry is only alive today because no government on earth will regulate it out of existence. The government has the power but will not use it,so if you are waiting for them to introduce draconian measures to whip the food industry into shape, then it is most likely that you will see a pig fly first,which considering the Frankenstein tendencies of the food industry is a distinct possibility.

20 Think about your food budget,because you are used to spending £100 per week, that amount should not be set in stone,if you check your purchases,you should be able to reduce or even increase your bill,if you were so inclined. If you lost your job today,you would have a serious incentive to get that figure down.
The more processed the food you buy,the higher the price of your weekly shop.
A trolley full of processed unhealthy wonders will cost considerably more than a trolley of raw materials to be prepared and cooked yourself. Cooking from scratch,you will get better value for money,a 1 kg bag of potatoes could stretch to 3 meals.,a whole fresh chicken is definitely a 2 meal job, possibly 3 if you use leftovers to make soup or toss them into a salad.

Question:
Do you spend more time on scrutinizing the prices on goods on Ebay or Amazon than your food budget?

21 Buying good food at decent prices and getting real value for money is great,but who has your back? Who is watching out for your interests? The food industry? Hell no!,they are looking for the cheapest suppliers to provide products that can be charged at the most they can get. All other considerations are rescinded as long as they aren't breaking the law or indulging in practices,that will result in bad publicity,a falling share price and shareholder displeasure.

The government is incapable,unwilling and always acts after the horse has bolted from the stable. In all fucking honesty,it is up to you. The government will not legislate against the food industry as they have done,against the tobacco business. Even though the food industry has probably done and will do more damage to human health than the tobacco industry ever did. As a result of toothless and spineless government policies,the food industry is feeding its customers to death. If the food industry had been allowed to draft government food policy,they couldn't have done a better job at creating lame policies that end up protecting their interests.

22 The only way for the food industry to survive profitably,is the use of their most effective weapon:retailers, especially in the form of supermarkets,who can:
Make you eat more than you should, with their numerous special offers.
Pay less than you should(think of alcohol prices or cheap fried fast food meals).
Buy more than you need with their built in convenience features such as easy use free car parks,large shopping trolleys,restaurants,post offices,extended opening hours and pharmacies.
All these aspects encourage you to stay longer in their stores,take for example,extended supermarket opening hours,these are not for their customers benefit,you no longer have,any excuse not to indulge every whim,no matter how fleeting, fancy a steak sandwich with chips at 1am,washed down with a cold bottle of Fosters,no need to ignore that desire,the supermarkets never close. Well apart from that legislated twilight zone between 4pm Sunday afternoon and Monday morning, even the supermarket god needs to rest.

23 When will the government be forced to take effective action? when we finally elect a government that does not fear or need the favours of the food industry,secondly, when the government gets a spine and admits that self regulation will never work,letting the food industry regulate itself is like putting a chocoholic in charge of a chocolate factory.
The food industry does not do self harm.
As more people are now dying from diet related illness than any other disease,the free will issue must be put aside, the government must step in step and introduce regulation. It needs to decide that the health of the people is more important than looking after their friends in the food industry,being accused of being a nanny state, future employment or being influenced by lobbies.

People have been allowed to make their own choices and look where it has got us,super sized children,super obese adults,reduced life expectancy,massive burden on the health services and the explosion in bariatric medicine.

It is obvious that against relentless advertising,cheap prices,ease of access,tasty filling quick fast foods and mini buckets of soft drinks,our self discipline has withered up and died of shame.

It is sad to admit that,we have lost the battle with our greed and desires,we never stood up against the providers of all this junk food,we did not vote with our wallets and refuse to purchase their products,we did not limit our consumption of their products to infrequent occasions.

The only time our mouths stop eating is when we are sleeping. We never questioned how on earth was all this food was provided so cheaply,we rarely questioned the ingredients ,as long as it did not poison us or make us ill at the first bite.

We forgot that too much of anything was bad, how in gods name,can drinking a litre of fizzy soft drink, with ingredients like sugar,colouring,phosphoric acid, flavourings,potassium sorbate and dimethyl dicarbonate, regularly be good for anybody? Because it is approved,legal and generally regarded as safe does not mean that it is right or sensible.

We overlooked the fact that if we de skilled ourselves of kitchen expertise,there would be hell to pay. It takes time and effort to cook a meal from scratch, time and effort that will erase any fleeting hunger pangs,but with the introduction of the microwave into homes and with it microwavable snacks and foods,coupled with the growing illusion that we do not have time to cook, we lost the battle.

If we cannot pass our cooking expertise onto our children,then their food choices are in the hands of amoral profit hungry companies.

We abandoned common sense,almost stopped drinking plain water and guzzled down ever increasing larger amounts of sweet,colourful,fizzy soft drinks.

Another battle was lost as the food manufacturers poured high fructose corn syrup into almost every processed food in sight,we just gobbled up all their products,you look at at label of ready made tomato pasta sauce,see sugar in it,do you say what the fuck? What is sugar doing in there? I don't sprinkle sugar onto my home made spaghetti bolognese,get the fuck out of my kitchen! No, you meekly accept it and you just follow instructions to stir the sauce constantly,so the sugar does not burn at the bottom of the pot.

We ate ourselves into this disaster, with political correctness abounding, do gooders making excuses for the victims,blaming others,it was nobodies fault,go to any GP practice or watch any television program featuring the obese(there are plenty) ,the fat are treated as victims,nobody dares say,you are in this sorry position because you could not stop eating and when you ate,you ate all the wrong stuff and you ate too much of it.

How in the hell did you not think that eating processed meals, takeaways every day,washed down with soft drinks, would not fuck up your life?

When you got to 15 stone did you not think that you ought to take action as you soared above your ideal weight? instead you ate even more,super glued your ass to the sofa all the way to 17 stone,your doctor did his best to reverse the position,but you ignored him and soon hit 25 stone,now you are house bound,depressed and still eating to 30 stone,in constant need of the big body squad.

You live in a democracy,you have the right to eat what you like,when you like,how much you like and how often you like but you better be prepared for the consequences.

On the other hand,we know those bastards in the food industry are selling crack cocaine passing as food but they did not force feed you. They offered temptation but where was your will power?

They sold it but you took yourself down to the shops,brought the stuff and scoffed it down on a regular basis,possibly even every day. You knew it was wrong but you made excuses to yourself,along the lines of:

"Its my treat"

"I haven't had it for a while" (you did last week)

"I don't drink or smoke"

"I know its naughty"

"It's the weekend"

"It makes me happy"

"There was nothing else around"

"It's quick"

The food industry is not your friend,its function is to sell profitable,addictive concoctions of fat,sugar and salt disguised as food to keep its shareholders happy,all other considerations are secondary.

You ate yourself to super obese all by yourself.

As long as you were not held down and force fed till you were obese then you must take ALL of the responsibility for your situation

The government will not help you,those jokers cannot even get the companies to pay tax in the first place

And if you want to reverse the situation,its all up to you,society will just adjust to your size by providing,stronger furniture,larger clothes sizes,tougher hospital equipment to bear your weight,careers in the bariatric industry,employment for builders to build suitable home improvements,tougher ambulances to carry you to hospital. The pharmaceutical industry will be rubbing its hands in glee at the profits it will make from the numerous drugs prescribed to you. Help yourself,other wise in this politically correct society,hardly anyone wanting to keep their job,is going admonish you about your weight and lifestyle. All you will get,is enablers who help you survive not change for the better.

24 Eating! what is it all about?

Food is sexy,

I eat out of boredom,

I am unhappy,I eat,

I am depressed,I eat,

Lets celebrate,lets eat

We lost,lets eat

We won, lets eat

I'm tired,I need to eat

I feel unloved,I'm eating

Its your birthday,bring in the cakes
I am loved,I'm eating
I am lonely, I'm eating
I love going to Nando's
I never drink water.
I am fat,eating makes me happy.
My partner no longer fancies me,I'm eating.
My marriage has gone to the dogs,food makes me happy.
I am too thin,I need to eat
I am too fat,eating makes me happy
I've just been dumped,where's the chocolate?
I live for my Chinese every Friday.
"Nothing tastes as good as skinny feels"
I hate my life,love my food
I hate my job,food makes me happy
I hate animal cruelty,I am a vegetarian
Just like my mothers
I deserve a treat,lets go to McDonald's for lunch.
I love a medium rare steak
I love to eat
I hate eating
Food is better than sex
That was great shag,lets eat.
Nobody loves me,where the Carte D'Or ?
Meat is murder
Cows are sacred
Pork is unclean
Its against my religion
I am a vegan
I love chocolate
I hate Brussels sprouts
I can't wait for the McRib to come back.
Drink and be merry
I hate alcohol
I couldn't resist
Lets get pissed
I'm dying for a glass of chilled Chardonnay
I'm gasping for a pint of ice cold cider
Its a lovely summer day,lets have a Barbecue
Lets celebrate,pop a cork
I'm anorexic
I need a treat,I need some chocolate
That looks good,lets have some.
Free of artificial flavours,colours and preservatives
Good for children
You've lost weight,you look great,sexy.
Just got paid,lets have a treat.

ITS NOT ABOUT THE MONEY, ALL EATING IS EMOTIONAL.

25Watch the ads. Every food advertisement on your television has slim people living the good life,however on the streets ,there are increasingly large numbers of overweight and obese people walking about. What are food advertisers trying to tell us?

Eat suggested portions of our products as clearly indicated on the packaging,live a healthy active life,combined with a balanced diet and you won't put on weight?

or

Just buy our products and you will look like this,great,sexy,slim and healthy.

or

see our ads packed with great looking slim people who consume our products,the fact that you can only shop at big and large clothing stores online has nothing to do with us.

Finally;

Its a free society,do what you like,no one has the right to tell you what to do,how much you should weight, who wants to live in nanny state,telling you what you can and cannot eat? we are just telling you about our fantastic products, how much,and how often you consume them is totally your choice.

But just check, the streets,your work place,buses,trains and hospitals and see the damage their products have wreaked on the population. Whose fault is it that 50% of Britons are over weight? or that 26% are classed as obese? The food industry?

for producing addictive crack cocaine disguised as irresistible food or us for lacking any kind of self control?

Is it our fault for consuming too much of their products ? but that cheese stuffed crust pizza is just so moreish,that handmade cupcake looks so delicious.

People are suffering from all manners of illnesses brought on, from overconsumption of products advertised by beautiful slim people. Have you ever seen an fat person in a chocolate bar advertisement? have you ever seen a true chocoholic who is slim?

That should convince you to leave your money in your wallet and watch what you buy.

26 Making sensible healthy food purchases is preferable to:
Diet Disasters
Health destroyers
Life expectancy reduction
Waist expanders
Scale busters
Two seat backsides
Wearing black to hide your bulk
Coronary inducers
Diabetes bringers
Stroke inducers
Tight clothes
Constant breathlessness

Chicken wings
Pot bellies
Godzilla thighs
Wobbly bits
Health professionals lecturing you (which can be ironic as they may not be pictures of health themselves)
Hospital visits
Pill Popping
Adverse side effects from daily pill popping
Health Specialist visits
Wearing sports clothing,such as tracksuits and jogging bottoms to hide your bulk, besides they are the only comfortable clothes you can get.
Fat kids
Early graves
Limited movement
Unable to stand the sight of yourself in the mirror;is all that heartbreak,depression and pain, worth eating a whole packet of Mr Kipling's French Fancies,washed down with a 2 litre bottle of Coke?

All of the above start with your food purchases,its your money spend it wisely or it will seriously fuck you up.
Buy the right foods,at the right quantities and eat a sensible amount.

Simples.

But

We all know its not as *simples* as that,but in the long term,only you and your nearest and dearest will suffer the consequences of eating so much fatcrap. And to be honest,food without any nutritional value,that ruins health and shortens your lifespan can only be described as fatcrap which is rubbish,deadly rubbish.

The company boss who manufactured the salt ridden snack,that helped to increase your blood pressure that led to your stroke,will retire to a tropical island with a great pension and the best medical care available on earth. Hell, Fred Goodwin fucked up BIG TIME and still walked off into the sunset with a taxpayer funded pension of
£342,500 a year after RBS lost £24.1 billion in 2008.

The supermarkets,you brought the fatcrap from, will continue to trade successfully long after you died of an heart attack caused by making the wrong food choices in their stores.
Tesco founded 1919
Sainsbury's founded 1869
Morrisons founded 1899
Asda founded 1949
Waitrose founded 1904
Aldi founded 1913
Lidl founded 1930

The feckless government that failed to protect you from the "profit at all costs" food industry will mercilessly tax your children and grandchildren to fund the escalating health costs involved in looking after your sorry ass,when you are afflicted by all kinds of diet related illnesses in your later years.

I have said it before and I'll say it again but in the long term,only you and your close ones will suffer the consequences of eating so much rubbish.

This is a true story.

Word.

Caveat Emptor.

27 For all their faults,all their marketing,promotions,bogofs,celebrity endorsements,addictive tasty food,cheap bargains,cheap booze,attractive superstores,convenience,ubiquity,opening hours,free parking,value added ranges,range of choice,discounts,loss leaders,vouchers, freebies,super sized offers etc.
The food industry does not hold a gun to your head,forcing you to hand over your money. Caveat Emptor will always apply.

Get some back bone,decide to make your own shopping choices,free of any outside influence.

28 The shopping trip to the supermarket, your purchases are killing you or not....... eventually.
Are you buying slow acting poison or life enhancing healthy food?

Its your money,do not choose.....poorly.

29 Food:only buy what you need.
Don't waste it,
Don't chuck it away,
Try this experiment, next time when food shopping,use cash instead of plastic. The psychological effect of handing over so many bank notes will encourage you to spend less of them. Using debit and credits cards is a subtle method to get you to increase your spending,after all you are only limited by your bank balance or credit limit not by the cash in your hand ,remember the days when you had to leave items behind because you didn't have enough money at the till. Now everybody just goes over budget,that is,even if you have one.

After all how can you monitor,something you cannot see,all you know is a certain figure has been deducted from your account. An invisible transaction,it sure is convenient but cashless transactions inevitably make you spend more.

You are not limited by the cash in your wallet, but your bank balance,so take advantage of all those special offers being thrown your way,which why they are there in the first place.

As we now live in the cashless age,the only limits to your spending are the limits you place on yourself.

30

We are what we think.

Your focus determines your reality

You are the result of your thoughts

We become what we think about

What ever your mind,can conceive and believe,it can achieve.

Our thoughts are the cause of every condition in our lives.

So DO YOU think about your food choices or not?

Are you just a passive consumer of what ever shite is passed your way? are you like a sheep that eats grass chewing,shitting,chewing and shitting?

Does your life run along the following lines:

open fridge,get food
put in microwave
put in mouth
dump in toilet

open freezer,get food
put in microwave
put in mouth
dump in toilet

open fridge,get food
heat on cooker
put in mouth
dump in toilet

open freezer get more food
put in oven
put in mouth
dump in toilet

get more food from supermarkets
put in freezer
put in microwave
put in mouth
dump in toilet

Every damn day,living a food obsessed life,avoiding healthy food, exercise and an active lifestyle.

31 Mastication

Chew slowly,chew each mouthful 20 times,stop gobbing food down like a hungry dog. eat slowly,chew slowly you will feel satisfied quicker,eating less,saving money. simples.

Speed eating,inhaling,wolfing it down,binge and mindless eating,are a major cause of weight gain.

When you speed eat, a packet of digestive biscuits,you would have over ridden all signals from your brain that you were full or sated after eating only 3 biscuits.

All the unchewed food in your belly is causing constipation,bloating,flatulence, cramps,diarrhoea and even insomnia,in short making you feel ill,lethargic and constantly unwell.

Eat slowly,take your time,nobody is taking your food away,there are tons of the cheap stuff about,in fact they are even shipping and flying it in from far off exotic locations only to throw it away because it does not look right.

32 You are tripping over hundreds of food sellers,Tesco local,Sainsbury's express,fried chicken kebab shops,sandwich shops,supermarkets,snack shops,coffee shops,burger restaurants,fish and chips shops,Chinese,Indian takeaways,cake shops,pubs the list and choice is endless. At every price range from the 99p burger to a fillet steak dinner at the Ritz,this wide ranging availability and convenience is a wallet emptier and health ruiner.

33 Step up and buy your own personalised ailment. Ladies,Gentlemen and Children,step up and move closer,here is your very own opportunity to get your own ailment,why be healthy and fit? why eat like a Tibetan monk,where is the fun in that? Self control? don't be soft.

Self discipline? what does that mean?

Exercise? Don't be daft.

Jogging? It's cold outside,

5 portions of fruit and vegetables? What am I,a rabbit?

Self control? Long time dead.

Step up,open your wallets,buy all the fat crap foods you love and enjoy,put a mortgage down on your own personal illness,enter the world of roller coaster health changes,pop tons of pills,take endless hospital tours, visit your doctor on a regular basis, here is the chance to take sick days off your boring job and still get paid! Take a tour of various NHS facilities,try and test its services,have a procedure done see what all the debate is about. Is it a great service? will it save your life? or is it just a big fat target for politicians,newspapers and commentators?

Here is the chance to get big,an excuse to go clothes shopping,avoid boring and repetitive exercise.

Just imagine,all that reckless eating of high calorie junk food and you never know what illness is coming your way, everybody likes surprises? it could be diabetes,cancer,stroke,coronary disease,PMS,food poisoning,headaches,cardiovascular disease,osteoporosis,high blood pressure,celiac disease,IBS,acne,depression,hypertension,cholesterol,sleep apnea,allergies,liver damage and so on and so forth,the choice is varied and unlimited. Step up and don't miss this once in a lifetime opportunity.

Which disease are you buying on a weekly mortgage basis?,this time we are using mortgage based on its French origins:Death contract.

We are what we eat,health sapping ailments are what you should expect,if you do not curb spending on fatcrap foods,which are certainly tasty but have zero nutritional value,in fact to save your life you would be better off setting fire to your money.

Question:
What is the difference between the high fat,high sugar,high salt western diet and famine?

None,they will both kill you....... Eventually.

Selah

34 When is a sale not a sale? a bogof is not a bargain unless you normally purchase the item. If you buy cornflakes every week,and this week there happens to a promotion in the form of a bogof or 33% more,then for you it is a real deal,as you are actually getting more for the same amount of money. Offers on your standard purchases are great deals,but any offer that makes you spend more, is only taking money from you. If it is not on your shopping list then it is a money taker.
The same applies to reduced goods,it is only worth buying,if it is a replacement for a more expensive item.
 Very few people save up to buy products,so sales are no longer value for money items. All these promotions,are you really saving or increasing your spending under the pretence of making savings. The rule to follow is; more for the same money or the same quantity for less money.

35 Everyday is not Christmas food shopping,when you chuck items into the trolley regardless of the cost or health considerations. Such carefree behaviour is fine once a year,but your weekly shop should be a study in discipline,not an excuse to load up the trolley with all kinds of nonsense that will end up in the dustbin,expand your waist,clog up your arteries and increase your blood pressure. Money wasted. Health fucked up.

36 Try fasting,to cleanse your digestive system. There are numerous ways to indulge in this healthy activity.

ADF- Alternate day fasting:
Eat and drink like a member of parliament on Monday
Nibble like a supermodel on Tuesday, a bread and water kind of thing.
On Wednesday,feast like a prince but on Thursday, its back to the meagre rations.

5.2 fasting
Feast like a male breakfast show presenter for 2 days
Eat like a female breakfast show presenter for 2 days,500 calories per day.

It might be harder to believe,in these days when we never stop eating,but fasting for long periods will not kill you. Trust me,you will not die from hunger. Fasting will help you detoxify and rest your digestive system, besides like all things in life,eating,fasting,drinking,spending,fucking and sleeping are best done in moderation.

37 World of waste. Yanks throw away 40% of food they buy,32% of food purchased in UK is binned.
The 3rd world wastes food due to inadequate storage facilities,the western world wastes food because they have too much of it.

WTF!

How did we come to this?

38 Slow down,you are not in a shopping or eating competition! Unless you are training to go on Man vs Food or undertaking serious training to be a competitive eater,why do you eat so much? and so fast? Why buy so much food?
Why do you make frequent trips, to buy the super-sized meals from fast food outlets (calling them restaurants is an insult to food,probably factory outlet is more apt,as almost everything they sell has come off a factory line)
Why do you like going to the "all you can eat" buffet restaurants?,why heap so much food on your plate? they aren't an exercise in taste, textures or balance of ingredients but to excess. Nobody ever goes to one of those places looking for haute cuisine,but for the chance to eat themselves silly. There is simply no wisdom or benefit in overeating,what do you get from it? apart from a bloated uncomfortable stomach and inevitable straining exercise in the toilet.
Stop now! Hands up! back away from the special fried rice,you are already full,you know that if you force yourself to finish the food on your plate and make another trip to the food counter,you will feel like a balloon about to burst for hours afterwards. And of course the weight gained from this greedy feast will soon manifest itself on your waist,thighs,arms,face,legs etc. etc.

Why do you do this to yourself?

Why do you have to eat a whole packet of chocolate digestives? were you not aware that you can eat 2 or 3 biscuits,stop and put the rest away for another day? the biscuit tin was created for this purpose. the borrowers are not waiting to steal your left overs away. No one is going to snatch your chocolate hobnobs away, so please stop inhaling a 500g packet in one sitting.
Do you need to finish that 2 litre stomach bloating,sugar laden bottle of fizzy drink in one go? free healthy zero calorie water is available from the nearest tap,in case you have forgotten.
Regular guzzling down that 4 pack of beer in one sitting, will stay on your waist until you are dead and buried or your GP is prescribing metformin for your newly diagnosed type 2 diabetes or insomnia inducing statins for cholesterol.

So once again I ask you,if you are not a competitive eater,or preparing to trek to the North pole,why do you buy so much,to eat so much? If you don't rein in your mouth,there are people queuing up to make money off you,when the consequences show up in and on your body.

By the way your kids are watching and learning from you,ready to pick up the baton,after you have died from diet related diseases. As they only learned to eat the same crap that killed you,if you never taught them to eat well,who will? Who are you counting on to do your job? TV,schools,the government,celebrity chefs or the food industry?

39 Selah : Is the global food business in all its forms ,the most destructive,deadly and corrupt force on the planet?
Oxygen giving rain forests cleared for cattle rearing
Government subsidised cheap corn syrup aiding the obesity epidemic
Endless diet related illnesses
Impact of junk food on children's health
melamine milk
Mad cow disease
Water bulked chicken and pork
The rise and rise of the food scientist.
Battery farming
Animal welfare
Food wastage
Farm and food subsidies
Famine
All conquering supermarkets reducing variety of shopping outlets and choice
All conquering supermarkets imposing lower prices on their suppliers
Food industry sourcing food from the cheapest suppliers from all around the world as a result they get horse meat instead of beef.
Food chain related illnesses such as salmonella.

How has it come to this? how has a necessity created so much evil? And your money supports it. You are what you buy. As long as you keep on demanding cheap food,
there are consequences,that come along for the ride.

40 The basic foodstuffs are the best,there is nothing new under the sun,nothing new has been discovered. All we have now, are variations,creations,combinations, aberrations,copies of the same old stuff, rolling off the production line at the mad scientists factory.
There aren't any new foods,the basic foodstuffs of today are the same as 100 years ago, in fact the choice has got narrower,most likely due to supermarket economics. Years ago we had much more varieties of fruit and vegetables to choose from,now price,longevity and looks being the main deciding factors. The basic untouched foodstuffs of veg,meat,poultry and fish are still some of the best things you can eat. There isn't any thing wrong with grilled chicken and steamed vegetables. It is all the valued added precooked,chilled,frozen monstrosities that are dangerous and deadly.

After all there isn't much you can do to screw up just one ingredient.
A sprinkling of salt and pepper on a roasted chicken,equals a delicious
meal,with no additives apart from that fed to the chicken to make it grow
faster,heavier and be disease free but that is a matter for another day.

41 Not all new products are great,has it never occurred to you that despite
thousands of new products launched daily,the space in the supermarket
shelves stay the same. So don't be tempted by that "new" label. It ain't new
,its just another godforsaken
temptation created by food scientists and marketing experts,to coax more
money out of your pocket. A perfect example is a certain cream cheese
spread mixed with chocolate.

42 Get Smart
Get yourself a food education,if you can learn to use social media then you
should be to find out about the the food products you buy.

* How are they grown?

* Where in the world, is it grown?

*How many air or sea miles has it clocked up to get to your gob? Like
Scottish cod,shipped to china for skinning and boning,then shipped back.

* Is it grown in soil or hanging from a tree?

* Who farms it? multinationals,cooperatives, farmers or children?

*Are the animals slaughtered humanely or are they terrified before they are
killed?

*What is in the food? beef,chicken,pork,horse meat or unknown from the
cheapest supplier?

*What the hell are those unknown items on the ingredients list? carmine?
xanthan gum? gelatin? sorbitol? phosphoric acid? carrageenan?
polydimethylsiloxane?,why are they in our food? What the fuck are they doing
in our food? Did you know that some processed foods can have up to 60
ingredients? When a food product has a combined total of 60 ingredients, you
know that nature and the farmer have abandoned food production to the food
scientists.

*Are chickens kept in filthy,stinking horrible conditions before they are
killed,cleaned,nicely packaged, and sold to you 3 for £10. Can any animal be
humanely reared to be sold at such a low price?

* Who was the bright spark,who discovered that it was extremely profitable to
inject chicken,ham and bacon with water and charge us by the weight for the
privilege? Which is probably why they can afford to sell 3 for £10

* The more pertinent question is,why the government has allowed the food industry to sell us water disguised as food ?

* Where the hell in Europe did that diced or minced beef come from? Is it really beef?

*Do children in the developing world have to forgo school or childhood,so that the western world can get relatively cheap food to eat itself to death and even waste half of it?

* Is getting food,cheap your main priority,all other considerations rescinded?

* Are people in the so called third world, toiling in horrible conditions to bring you your favourite products at rock bottom prices,? over a thousand people died in a building collapse in Bangladesh, so cheap seekers in the west could purchase clothes at ridiculously low prices.

* Is the food industry operating a "don't ask,don't tell policy? You as the customer will not hear,see or speak no evil as long as you can get a cheap shopping basket.
May be it is karma working,that cheap basket of food is ruining our health and shortening our lives.

What is your money contributing to the world?

In the long run,greater food knowledge leads to better food choices,which in turn,can heighten health awareness.

You should know what the effect of every mouthful of food you take,has on your body. Is it killing me slowly or sustaining me ?

43 Food shopping is not,and should never be a leisure activity.
If the weekly food shop,is the highlight of your life then you need to get a new one.
Seeing this as leisure activity to be anticipated,then you are most likely shopping with your guard down and will fall for all the usual gimmicks. The lighting,colourful packaging,attractive displays,lack of windows,clocks to make you lose sense of time,relaxing atmosphere(sometimes) and free parking,are all designed to make you chill out and spend yourself happy.

Essentially you are a lab rat in a carefully constructed maze. It is no accident that every supermarket in the world has the same interior layout:race track aisles, attractive displays,the easy parking facilities,in short, you are shopping in the midst of some carefully applied science of human behaviour.

44 Don't believe the hype? Are discounts really bargains? or are they mind fucks,retail traps or confusions cons on an "Inception" level.
Such as when 2 smaller packs at 90p are cheaper than the large one at twice the size at £2 or the pack size and price has not diminished but the contents inside have.

45 You still have choice,please exercise it. You still make choices on everyday decisions,such as which film to watch in the cinema,clothes to buy,insurance to take,your next mobile phone but mysteriously once you cross into the realm of supermarket world,your ability to choose becomes seriously impaired,you shop in a daze,dodging trolleys and picking up special offers. Its only when you get home ,unpack your shopping then you start to wonder, why did I buy this? why did I buy 2? how did I spend over £100,what do I have to show for it? What the fuck did I spend my money on?

It is this shopping in a semi daze,guard down approach,that makes so many of us buy health ruining fatcrap food and drinks,which are always on offer.

46 Abundance in the western world is killing us,we suffer from numerous self inflicted ailments and are dying from too much not lack.
W T F!
Dying from living the good life,simply because we eat too fucking much and never allow ourselves to suffer hunger pangs or even go hungry. Our stomach never rumbles with hunger. Everyday is a christmas feast in the western world,the worlds poorest grow our food,build our gadgets,toys,furniture,manufacture our clothes. We have been living off the fat of the land of the poor and now it is killing us.
Now enter the temple of doom:supermarkets,we have tea from India,coffee from Kenya,oranges from Israel,raisins from California,apples from South Africa,wine from France, toys made in China,clothes from Vietnam,salami from Italy,shelf stacker's from Poland,cleaners from Africa,chicken from Holland,beef from Brazil, horse meat from the EU.

Somebody is getting seriously wealthy from all this, surely not the poor sods who make the stuff in the west or the cheap seekers in the west, who do you think?

We can get what we want,when we want,eat what ever we desire,we are not limited or restricted by distance,season,price,war,technology,famine,natural disaster or time.
The feast just goes on with an unlimited, buffet choice, If continue like this,we will eat ourselves into extinction.
We also have the gadgets,technology to extend the shelf life of our foods. Irradiate the tomatoes to last until people live on the moon. Unlike the poor in the third world,who can only eat fresh seasonal produce, as they don't have storage facilities and eat the basic natural foods because they cannot afford expensive processed rubbish.
Their food choices are great,fresh, healthy but what kills them is famine,poor medical services,dirty water and war, factors often out of their control.

On the bright side for them, at least their food choices aren't killing them,like us .

47 Is your self control so weak as to be non existent? do you employ any of the following concepts in your life?

Self control
Self discipline
Abstinence
Goal setting
Avoidance
Forbearance
Frugality
Fasting
Moderation
Refraining
Self denial
Calorie counting
Restraint
Sobriety
Temperance
Giving up
Refusal
Rejection
Relinquish
Restriction
Sacrifice
Withhold
I'll pass
No thank you
Not for me
NO!

48 Fat parents,Fat kids,Fat grandchildren,fat great grandchildren, Fat
generation, that should be enough to put a chill down your spine.
You cannot cook to save your life,your children will probably never learn to
even boil an egg. Consequently you are putting their health into the hands of
people who put 10 teaspoons of sugar into a can of soft drink,gave us horse
meat instead of beef,
hydrogenated fat,turkey twizzers, vegetable fat instead of cocoa butter in
chocolate bars. Carry on at your peril.

49 You can never be too thin.(at least try to put it to the test)

50 This may help:
If cannot tell the source or origin of a food by looking at it,then it is bad for
you; simples.
Cow-beef steak-burger
chicken-drumstick-nuggets
fish-steak-fish-fingers
pork-chop,ribs-sausage or bacon.
The final transformation always has added undesirables.
Stick to unprocessed foods,which are better value for money that their
processed counterparts. Processed foods should be avoided as much as
possible, a pork chop is inherently better than a sausage which has added

fat,rusk and salt plus other additives added to it. another example is meatballs,get some mincemeat,add some spices to it,salt,finely diced onions,roll then into balls,fry them or cook them in the oven,natural meatballs but purchase frozen ones or processed ones,the ingredients list excluding beef is as long as your arm. Make the transformation yourself.

51 Are you too fat to fly?
Are you too fat to walk?
Are you too fat to sleep soundly?
Are you too fat to bend down?
Are you too fat to work?
Are you too fat to fuck?
Are you too fat to under go an operation?
Are you too fat to leave your house?
Are you too fat to drive?
Are you too fat for your furniture?
Are you too fat to take your children to the park?
Are you too fat to buy your clothes from the high street?
Are you too fat to go to a gym?
Are you too fat to walk your children to school?
Are you too fat to visit the place that played a part in making you fat;supermarkets?
Are you too fat to walk into any fast food outlet,without people staring at you,thinking " you really don't need to be here"?

Question: what do you think,you need to do?

52 What are you spending your money on?
Soft drinks,fruit juices,smoothies- Obesity in a bottle
Crisps,chocolate bars,breakfast bars,biscuits- Obesity in a pack
Sugary breakfast cereals- Obesity in a box.
Hamburger meals-quick served obesity
Fried chicken shops-fast fried obesity
Chinese and Indian-take away obesity
Carefully consider your food purchases,especially the calorie jacked meals that contain in a single serving,a days calorie requirement. Think about all the effort,you have to expend in order to burn off,all the calories from eating those French fries.
Caveat Emptor will always apply.

53What are you spending your money on? part 2.
Save yourself,curb your spending on obesity causing foods,buying that crap,means that you are using your hard earned money to buy foods that can ultimately ruin you and your child's health.
You as a parent are primarily responsible for making sure that your child eats healthily,not the school,not the food manufacturers or the even the government.
So let me ask you these questions;
Is your child overweight?
Who over fed them?

Who brought all the fizzy drinks?

Who paid for all the takeaways?

Who went to the supermarket and brought burgers,chips,pizza,sausages,cakes chocolates,crisps,biscuits,soft drinks?

Who went to the supermarket and did not buy water,fresh fruit and vegetables?

Who allowed them to sit in front of the computer or television for hours, hiding from the sun,avoiding fresh air and strenuous activity?

Who somehow failed to notice that the child had to have bigger school uniforms?

Who failed to notice that the child was growing sideways and not upwards?

Who neglected to show them a life of exercise,sensible healthy eating?

Who drove the children to school,when they could easily walk?

Who gave into their demands for fatcrap?

Who was the parent who failed to notice that their child was getting fatter than them?

I'm sure it wasn't the people at number 10 but the parent in the mirror.

It is your job. Stop being a victim,take charge,take control,do not pass your responsibility onto someone else.

You created the fat child that you are looking at.

You can still undo your work.

Try not to purchase the ill health of you and your nearest and dearest.

This government WILL NOT BAN any foods that are overloaded with with fat,sugar and salt.

Once again with feeling, IT WILL NEVER HAPPEN. Let me repeat that, it will never happen.

It is your job not to buy the damn things in the first place.

The government has not yet banned deathly cigarettes,have they?

They have heaped taxes on them

Stuck large warnings on packets

Placed scary,explicit,frightening,and sometimes disgusting pictures on packets

Run anti smoking advertisements

Banned advertisements

Hid them from sight

Place age restrictions on them.

Although they shied away from putting them in plain packets

Yet people still smoke,what's up with that?

54 At this point of reading,do you still need a reason to reduce your spending on delicious,tasty,filling fat,salt and sugar laden danger foods.

Fatcrap in a word.

In late 2012,the lancet,reported that obesity now kills more people than hunger!

WTF! how did we come to this?

Non-communicable diseases such as diabetes,stroke and heart disease now kill more people globally than malnutrition,infectious diseases,maternal and childhood illnesses.

Overconsumption of high fat, high sugar,high salt processed foods combined with lack of exercise is wiping out people. This western lifestyle is being adopted all over the globe,especially by the younger generation,who will be hooked for life on this eat more than you need,move less that is required lifestyle.

So the whole world is slowly eating itself to death. (until that trillion dollar miracle pill arrives that helps stimulate significant fat loss without any side effects)

This situation is so fucked up,in a world where obesity is now killing more people than hunger,dying from starvation should be extinct,shouldn't it.

In a world where over consumption of food is causing more illness and death than any other factor. Nobody on this planet should suffer or die from lack of food.

How has it come to this?

55 Go teetotal. Think of how much you could save on abstinence from booze. Consider the health benefits,more energy,ability to focus and generally feeling better no more hangovers,blackouts,drunken rages,poor decisions,drunken sex,weight loss, no more money pissed away.

Quit smoking? don't even get me started,you are better off just putting a match to your money,at least you are not killing yourself at the same time.

56 Stick to unprocessed foods,they are cheaper and better for you,the shorter the ingredients list,the better the food.

On the other hand, a value beefburger contains a list of horrors,that you would never touch,if you really knew what you were eating.

Cheap food is really nutritionally poor ,with a sliver of original content and bulked up with cheap filler and enhanced with salt,sugar,fat and spices to make it edible(I mean tasty).

You might be saving money by buying them in the first place but you are also ruining your health and shortening your life span at the pretence of making savings you wont be around to enjoy.

You would be much better off buying the better,more expensive stuff and eating less of it. Steak instead of hamburger. one damn good steak a week than 2 nights of eating value burgers with their mystery contents.

Nearly all fatcrap foods are tasty and moreish which is why they keep being purchased and for many,they can never be substituted with fresh fruit or vegetables.

What would you rather eat? roast chicken and spinach salad or the latest burger meal from your nearest Mcfactory outlet.

Your answer to that question,will determine the course your future health will take.

Or possibly you really don't give a shit,maybe if you are living the good life,great partner,happy kids,big bank balance,flash car,great life prospects,fantastic career,its all good for you, you would never want it to end,so you would do everything within your power to keep the good times going,including eating healthy foods,exercising on a regular basis,living an active lifestyle.

On the other hand,if your life was miserable,with a job you hated,horrible kids,useless partner,no fucking prospects,clapped out car,why would you want to eat well to extend your miserable hopeless existence? you have a complete lack of self pride,what motivation could you possibly have to lead a healthy lifestyle? what is the fucking point of tiring yourself out with exercise and eating healthy boring food? Your situation is so fucked up, you are so miserable,desperately unhappy and feel trapped.

Very few things in your life, makes you happy or gives you pleasure like eating all those naughty foods. Consuming them makes you happy,the pleasure keeps the misery of your life at bay,until you look in the mirror. Food for you is not just sustenance,but a pleasurable addition,a high;that makes your

own personal unhappiness liveable.

Why motive could you possibly have,to extend your life? you might as well eat tasty crap that gives you pleasure,admittedly short lived . The NHS will try to keep you alive ,as long as possible despite your attempts to eat yourself to death.

The greatest strength of modern fast food is its consistency, (unlike chefs,the production line machines, never have an off day)it will deliver that same taste sensation time after time. Your life has its ups and downs but that Big Mac always delivers that mouth orgasm. Time after time,how could you resist that? What food tickles your g spot? that will always deliver a mouth orgasm?A cupcake? Chocolate? Indian? Chinese? Chocolate digestives? Mom's home made?

It sure as hell isn't fruit, vegetables or salad

Later you see all that damage in the mirror,you get depressed,only a bar of chocolate will alleviate your sadness and make you happy,another pleasurable mouth orgasm. The cycle starts again.

57

Don't be a supermarket snob,loyalty does not pay. If you normally shop at Fortnum and Masons or Waitrose,you are allowed to venture to the dangerous territories of Sainsburys and Tesco. And if you are feeling really adventurous,why not try the wild lands of Lidl,Aldi,Iceland and Farmfoods. Do your research,go where the bargains are,take advantage of each supermarkets strengths,Iceland and Farm foods have a great range of frozen foods but very limited on fresh fruit and veg. In fact your typical fresh veg&fruit section in a Tesco store dwarfs an entire Iceland store.

Aldi and Lidl have a great range of products which are considerably cheaper than the main brands and probably just as good,but you must be ready to endure long queues as staffing all their tills is not one of their top priorities which is why their products are cheaper.

Tesco,jack of all trades,one visit to their enormous "high street in a shed",you probably never have to go anywhere else,adequate and boring. Suits people who prefer to do all their shopping in one location.

Every supermarket has its benefits,learn to take advantage of them. Variety after all is the spice of life.

58 Statins,tight
clothes,cancer,breathlessness,depression,fatigue,metformin,visits to
hospitals,£7.90 prescription charges,painful knees,diabetes,heart
diseases,global warming,food miles,child labour,child obesity,wider plane
seats,bigger clothes,this is what you are really buying at the supermarket,if
your food choices are poor.
For every action,there is a reaction.

59 Dare I say it,Go veggie,try it,even if you decide that you can't live without
tearing into dead flesh,then cut down on the dead animals,watch 10 Disney
Pixar movies back to back,this will help. Jesting aside , you will save a
considerable amount of cash. You don't even need to buy the vegetarian
alternatives such as veggie burgers,sausages or quorn products. You can
even chop or mince vegetables to cook a veggie bolognese or chilli
concarne,try to go meat free for a day,a couple of days or even weeks,for
example no meat Mondays, creature free weekends,veggie wednesdays and
no animals before 6pm.

60 Use the manufacturers guidelines for portion control and servings,if it is a
four portion packet,then why in God's name are you finishing the whole pack
by yourself?.
When its all said and done,the food manufacturers are trying to play their
part(maybe half heartedly),pick up any food product,it will have portion
guidelines,calorie,sugar,fat and salt content.
Visit the titans of fast food; Mcdonalds,KFC and you will find on the tray paper
liner, the full nutritional information and allergy information on everything they
sell,which includes,kcal,protein,fat,carbs,fibre,salt,sugar and allergen
information. Even on their main display,it shows the recommended daily
calorie intake for men and women
and the calorie content of EVERY product on sale.
The information is there for us to read study and use by slowly backing out of
the outlet,but do we? Hell no,it is easier to eat a big mac meal everyday for
lunch and a 12 inch pizza for dinner and end up being portrayed as a victim of
the food industry,on one of the many television shows on obesity.

61 Greed is not good,at least when it comes to eating. Stop eating and back
away from
that whole packet of chocolate digestives.

There are no greedy thin people.

62 If you don't monitor your food shopping,you cannot manage it. how much
do you spend weekly?,have you brought the good stuff or an array of fatcrap?
Have you brought stuff you can cook yourself?
have you brought an array of ready made meals? which have amounts of
salt,sugar and fats which are out of your control.
Have you brought a trolley of real foods or laboratory created horrors?
Have you brought a trolley of salt,sugar and fat disguised as food?
How many calories were in the last meal you had?
Was the salt content within the recommended daily limit?

Do you know the daily calorie limits are?
In case you may have forgotten
Calories 2000 kcal
Sugar 90 grams
Fat 70 grams
Salt 6 grams

How many calories do you consume on a daily basis?

63The entire food industry makes money from you when you are eating their fatcrap products and putting on weight and consequently ruining your health.

The entire food industry makes money from you,when you are trying to lose weight and buying their low fat but high sugar,diet products.

The entire food industry makes money from you,when you make the decision to get healthy and buy their pro biotic,omega enriched, energy giving functional foods.

The drugs industry makes money from you,when you need to buy their products to deal with the ailments the food industry has inflicted on you.

The clothes industry makes money from you,every time you have to change your wardrobe to go up a size or a couple of sizes as the food industry has made you bigger.

The clothes industry makes even more money from you,if you have successfully slimmed down and need to change your wardrobe.

The clothes industry makes money from you,when you inevitably put on that lost weight again and have to buy another wardrobe.

The second hand clothes industry profits from buying all your clothes,you have built up from your weight going up and down, for £7 a kilo and selling them on for a massive profit.

The clothes industry makes money from you when you have to constantly buy bigger sizes for your transforming children. Its amazing how they seem to change size and shape in the blink of an eye.

The fitness industry makes money every time you pay the monthly subscription to your local health club to help improve your health, to combat the damage the food industry has inflicted upon you.

The fitness industry makes money from you,when under the delusion of making new year resolutions,you sign up to their health club and after a couple of weeks,you drop off the radar.

The government has to raise taxes from your earnings to fund the NHS,which is needed to treat the self inflicted victims of the food industry. If the political party seeking office, promises not to raise taxes during election time,then it will have to cut services that could help improve your health and probably save your life.

Celebrity chefs make millions from the collective pockets of those who buy their books, products and go to their restaurants.

The food industry makes money from you, when your children,now successfully hooked on their products,pester you to make purchases. Once your children are hooked, on fatcrap junk food,you so fucked.

Greedy business owners make money from your children,when they cynically decide to open a fast food takeaway near a school,which can give them a guaranteed lunch and after school trade.

Greedy business owners make money from you,when they decide to sell chips,pizza,chicken and burgers cheaper than school meals and offer larger portions as well. How many children can resist burgers,french fries,pizza and fried chicken?,can you?

The food industry makes money from you by selling take away fatcrap foods at such low prices that it seems cheaper and convenient than cooking yourself. Without any time spent in preparation,no waiting,no washing up,no hassle,you can get two pieces of chicken and chips with a canned drink for £1.99 and you are full afterwards.
Cheap and filling but a belly full of crap.

The food industry makes money from you when they flog BBQ kits,burgers,sausages and beer during sporting events which is ironic, as sports are all about abstinence,discipline and healthy eating. Lets not forget the heavily promoted belly blowing Christmas food shop.

The food industry makes money from you when you go to the cinema,theatre,stadium and find food prices set at rip off prices,as you have no choice and you cannot bring in your own food,you are forced over to hand over large wads of cash for over priced food. The food industry has never failed to take advantage of a captive audience.

The food industry makes money from you,when you choose to hear,see and speak no evil,chickens are reared in disgusting batteries for, you to buy 3 for £10. People in 3rd world countries living on less than a $1 a day are producing most of our coffee, fresh vegetables and fruit. It is probably the reason we can buy our food relatively cheaply,if food was as expensive as many people now say it is, it would probably be very difficult to become overweight.

Global warming is upped as planes fly in cheap globally sourced food. rainforest are cleared to raise cattle for cheap burgers.

You know this already,have heard it thousands of times but you remain quiet,you the cheap seeker.

The food industry has brought your conscience and silence for a cheap basket of your weekly shopping. The only way for you to obtain cheap goods is for another human being to be paid extremely low wages or non at all. What does that make you? a facilitator of human exploitation,a hundred years ago that was called slavery. We now have the modern low wage version,since slavery is out of the question.

The food industry makes money from you by selling products with cheap fillers with your full knowledge and thereby consent. frozen burgers have 60% meat content ,sausages can have 55% pork, pizza can have mock cheese topping,soya pieces,chicken nuggets can have 60% chicken,juice drinks can have 10% real juice,the rest is just cheap filler, you would probably refuse to feed your pet. You know this and still continue to buy the product,not demanding and be willing to pay for products with 100% original content. What are you,a cheap skate?

The food industry makes money from you due to your lackadaisical attitude,every major revealing food scandal is a storm in a teacup,the story breaks,followed by lots of outrage, government ministers talk about "lessons to be learned",the food industry changes what ever unsavoury practice they have been caught doing,with promises to do better in the future,eventually everybody soon calms down,forgets the scandal and goes back to the non stop feast.

When are you going to do the right thing? When are going to do something for yourself.
Everybody is making money from you,relying on your laziness and speak no evil attitude. When are you going to take action,or has eating so much fatcrap dulled your conscience.

How long were the following practices going on for until they were revealed and due to public disapproval were stopped?
Hydrogenated fats
Sudan 10
Mad cow
E.coli
Horse meat
GM foods
E numbers
Tainted milk in china.
All in pursuit of greater profit margins,it all about the money.

When the last tree is cut down
The last fish eaten
The last stream poisoned
And all food comes from the scientists lab

in order to cut costs
Cheap seeker you will realise that money cannot be eaten.

64 Save money,extend your life span,the meal combination from the past;
meat and two veg was the closest thing we had to the eat well,portion or diet
plate which shows the various types of foods,we should be eating and in the
correct portions. If you hate dieting or the sight of a cold salad makes you
shiver in disgust,or even hate eating healthily but deep down,seek a really
easy method to just eat right,then buy a portion plate,then shop and eat
according to its requirements.

65 Calories:
Men require 2500 calories daily
Women require 2000 calories daily
Teenagers require 2600 calories daily
Children require 1970 calories daily

So why the hell are you buying so much food?
Your fridge and freezer is completely stocked up,you have to force stuff in,just
to get
the door shut.
The cupboards are overflowing
Your belly enters a room before you do
Your clothes are tight
It is hard to get off the sofa
You cannot walk long distances
Your mouth never stops moving
You have over dosed yourself with treats
You are on first name terms with all the staff at your local takeaway
You still have your regular weekly takeaways despite the rising prices
Close to hand are all the takeaway menus for your local Chinese,Indian,pizza
and fried chicken shop.
You know by heart all their opening and closing times.
As soon as the takeaway answers the phone ,they know its you and know
what you are going to order before you can say a word.
Programmed into your phone's favourite contacts is the number of your
favourite takeaways.
In these days of the cashless society,you always have money ready for the
delivery driver.
Gentleman,looking straight down, you cannot see your dick due to your big
protruding belly. You can just about see your toes
You are always thinking of going on a diet.
You get depressed when you refuse to look at yourself in the mirror
You get even more depressed,when you do look at yourself in the mirror.
You are so unfit,your three year old child runs rings around you.
The health and safety officer at work recommends that you require a bigger
stronger chair.
Your tights are rubbing against each other.
You are considerably bigger than your partner.

Your children are fatter than you.

Your children cannot walk long distances or play sports.

The human resources manager is very familiar with your sickness record due to your never ending diet related illnesses.

Your colleagues are never surprised when you phone in sick.

You eat on the sofa,watching TV as a result eating more than required you are focused on the TV show hence ignoring the signals from your brain saying that you are full.

Your dining table no longer lives up to its name.

You always make sure that colleagues bring cakes to work for their birthdays.

Broken furniture in your house because you are simply too heavy.

Buying clothes online as the high street shops do not stock your size.

You always finish your massive takeaways as you cannot bear to throw it into the bin.

You do not stop eating when you are full.

You need a tablet sorter as your GP has prescribed so many pills for your diet related ailments.

Why do you buy so much when you need so little? consuming more than 2000 calories on a daily basis,will lead to excess weight.

Have we all fallen to victim to the illusion that we need to eat more food than we actually need? we are surrounded by food shops,supermarkets,adverts on the TV,on the internet,in magazines,newspapers and posters on the street. Is it any surprise that we think that we need to eat all the time. Open your weekend newspaper,it will have a food and drink section,with an article from some celebrity chef about their latest creation accompanied with some beautiful photographs,which make you salivate like Pavlov's dogs and excited enough to head for the kitchen to find a snack to satiate your hunger. Food is the new porn. And you know people cannot get enough porn or food.

66 Are you guilty?

Sweets and chocolates always in your bag?

Start every day with a fried breakfast? Or the modern version, McDonald's?

Start everyday with a muffin and a mini bucket of milky sugary expensive coffee?

Fallen for the spin that a super sweet breakfast bar or biscuit is more nutritious than a proper sit down breakfast,like a bowl of porridge?

Have a mini convenience store in you desk drawer at work?

Always finish a packet of biscuits in a sitting? You totally believe that once a packet is opened, it must be finished regardless of size,otherwise the manufacturers would have made it resealable.

You think that drinking plain water is unnatural.

Wash your curry down with fizzy soft drink or beer?

There is always a snack or chocolate bar in your bag?

 Head for KFC,McDonald's,when you damn well know that you should not. (anybody determined to eat well should never go near those places on a regular basis)

Is your only exercise,running upstairs to the bog?

Always out of breath?

Park next to the supermarket entrance to avoid walking too far?

Biscuits,chocolates,fatcrap foods are always in the house?
Cannot contemplate eating 1 portion of fruit or vegetables,not to talk of 5.
Throw out untouched fruit,salad and fresh vegetables,that have gone off?

67 Why don't you stay hungry,are you so desperate to eat,that you need to
snack in between meals,how about getting to the dinner table hungry like the
wolf?
Do you really need that arsenal of in between snacks?
But now we never stop munching,as a result we shop like we are stocking up
for the oncoming world war. And we tend to eat all we have brought.

Try this novel idea,eat only when you are hungry,really hungry.

The more crap you eat,the greater the likelihood that your latter years will be
spent on a merry go round of drug treatments and hospital visits. Wouldn't it
be great to remain ailment free in your old age,going about your
business,untouched by any diet related illness until you were 90,fell asleep
and did not wake up.
You passed away, simply because your time was up and not because,you
spent all your life dazzled by the food industry, ate too much of their product
and died of
a diet related illness due to your own lack of self control.
68
Buying the bad stuff and eating all you buy and you will inevitably have to
change your description to:
Obese
Super obese
Fat
Overweight
Big
Chubby
Chunky
Plump
Bariatric
Stout
Portly
Bulky
Large
Big boned
Extra large
Super sized
Pudgy
XXL
XXXXL
Tubby
Heavyweight
Super heavyweight
Lardy
Lard ass
Fat ass

Unfit
BBW
BBM
Plumper
Fatso
Heifer
Hog
Whale
Fatty
Blimp
Fat Cow

When you look in the mirror,what do you call yourself?

Beautiful?

Epilogue.

What can you do to help yourself?

It probably boils down to 2 issues
Key 1 Eating too much and too much of the wrong stuff. You can eat 5 pieces
of fruit and vegetables daily with no problem, its the chomping down of 5
donuts /cakes / chocolate bars and litres of fizzy soft drinks that will most
likely ruin your health.

Key 2 Moving too little; Your ass is stuck to the car seat,sofa and office chair.
You need to get active for extended periods of time. Walking from the car park
to the supermarket does not count.

Move one key downwards and move the other upwards to lengthen your life
and improve your health. Our primary concern here is key 1 as you are buying
too much and you eat everything you have brought. Maybe we listened too
well to our mothers who admonished us not to waste the food on our plates.

Stop buying things that take your fancy on the supermarket shelf,only to get
home,unpack your shopping,then wonder why you brought the thing in the
damn place. Also never go shopping hungry.

 Take no more crap! create your shopping at list at home and stick to it!
Any items missed off,can go onto the following weeks list,you won't starve
meanwhile and the supermarket will still be there packed to the rafters with
goodies.
Start a no fast food week in your house or a cook all your food fortnight. Limit
takeaways to emergency situations such as no food in the house (highly
unlikely).
Use twitter,facebook to start a national campaign based on home cooking.
Learning to cook,will help you take back control over what goes into your food
and make you less reliant on fattening factory output.

Get a petition going, set up a political party,start a riot!(joking) march to Downing street,demand that the feckless government take strong positive and changing action against the food industry in all its forms. Softly,softly has not worked,a take no prisoners attitude needs to be employed against the food industry until it is brought to heel. The all powerful collective of food retailers and manufacturers need to be hit with so much legislation,they will need to eat their own products for comfort.

Maybe the government should tackle car culture,people have become so lazy,they drive everywhere,including short distances that would take no effort to walk.
Those in power could consider making public transport free and place sky high taxes on unnecessary motoring.
Who knows,maybe this will get people out of their cars and back onto shanks pony.
A 20% tax on calorie jacked fast food and fizzy soft drinks should encourage people to reduce the amount of fatcrap they consume and hopefully change to healthier options. On the other hand increased taxes have hardly changed the behaviour of smokers,drinkers or drivers.

 This is an ongoing battle,you will probably never win the war,you will fall off the wagon and buy all kinds of tasty fatcrap,enjoy devouring it and feel guilty afterwards but dust yourself off,have no regrets,get back up and enter the fray once more.
When its all said and done, it is your responsibility to control what you eat,no one is coming to your rescue,this ain't no Hollywood movie. John McClane is not going to rescue you from the attack of the calorie monsters.
You have to be on guard all the time,sleeping with your eyes open and hand on your gun,(in reality your wallet).
Wage war with your most potent weapon,your hard earned cash,if you divert all your spending away from fatcrap foods and buy more healthy products,the money chasing food industry will have no choice but to provide you with what you want in order to earn their profit. To them it's all about the money, if tomorrow everybody in the world woke up vegetarian,the food industry will change course as soon as possible to meet the demand.

Apart from watching what you eat, getting fit and healthy,is not about being well off to pay for gym membership or having the time to exercise but just pure determination to do right for yourself.
As it says in the ad;Just do it:
Be determined to walk to work if the distance is less than 3 miles.
Be determined to get off the train or bus, one stop before you normally get off and walk the rest of the journey to your destination. Wake up earlier,if you have to.
Be determined not to watch that brain numbing reality programme with its fame hungry participants and take your pedometer for a long walk instead.
Those participants on reality television are trying to increase their income,you better sort yourself out,other wise that idiot will soon be able to afford a private

fitness tutor,whilst you are growing fat on the couch,watching the next bunch of idiots making their dash for fame and cash.

Be determined to cut down on your medication(seek your G P's advice first),tablets for blood pressure,cholesterol levels and blood sugar levels are chemical alternatives for doing the right thing,if you lived an active life,ate the right foods,it is unlikely that you will require a repeat prescription.

Be determined to stick to the eat well plate guide to portion size

Be determined to learn to say NO when you are offered a tempting snack when you are not hungry.

Be determined to stock up with products from the fruit and vegetable sections and not the obesity in a packet section.

Be determined to eat said fruit and vegetables and not feed them to the dustbin.

Be determined to limit the fast foods to one treat a month or give up them entirely,you won't be missing anything. It always tastes the same anyway,move on,nothing to see there.

Be determined to cook your own food with ingredients chosen by yourself.

Be determined to not let your children follow your unhealthy lifestyle.

Be determined to remember that your nutritional choices are far better than the previous generation but will probably have a shorter lifespan than them,if you continue to chose poorly.

Be determined to remember that this generation currently suffers and will continue to suffer from more diet related illnesses than any other since human history began.

Be determined to remember than overeating now kills more people than famine.

Be determined to remember that no matter how happy you are being overweight,you will definitely feel better being slimmer.

Be determined to get a pedometer and take it for a long walk,achieving at least 10,000 steps a day.

Be determined to remember than nothing tastes as good as thin feels.

Be determined to boldly go were you have never gone before and learn to become a cook or eat 5 portions of fruit and vegetables daily,drink water instead of fruit juice.

Be determined to boldly go where you have never gone before and learn to love the dreaded salad.

Be determined to tool up with the right gadgets and smart phone apps,such as scales,blood sugar, blood pressure monitors and walking boots.

Be determined to change your life into the direction you wish it to go.

Be determined to serve no master but your goals.

Be determined to get to achieve your goal, no matter what it takes.

Be determined to exercise on a regular basis

Be determined to learn to say no to sugar,salt and fat in its various disguises of chocolates,crisps,cakes,soft drinks,pizza the list of is endless.

Be determined to set short term and long term goals for your diet and health and make sure that you damn well reward yourself when you achieve them.

Be determined to always remember that your focus determines your reality.

To get something you have never had,you have to do something you have never done.

You are going to have to fight for your health.

It is our fault really, as soon as we de-skilled ourselves of kitchen abilities and became cheap seekers of food, the food industry stepped up to the plate and filled in the gap with very tasty,addictive and health ruining alternatives. Technology did the rest with the microwave in every home. With our de-skilling, we also abdicated our position of personal responsibility, especially the dictum that too much of anything is bad and caveat emptor. Even now with all the knowledge that we have,of the benefits of healthy eating, we still carry on chomping down the bad stuff regardless.

You are already obese,can hardly breathe,walk or fuck,yet you still carry your big self into a fast food restaurant and order,a burger,large chips,side and a large drink. For example,a large Big Mac meal that contains 1160 calories. 1160 calories,you do not really need. It does not take any effort for anybody to consume 3000 calories a day,if just one meal will provide over a thousand calories.

Yet the cause of your obesity is not really your fault? Get real!
Has your self discipline crawled down a hole and died of shame. You know that your middle name is unhealthy,but the easiest action to take is pop another cake into your mouth.
What kills.....eventually
Bad food kills
Fast food kills
Sugar laden food kills
Salty food kills
Greasy food kills
Cheap food kills
Junk food kills
Too much food kills
Too little food kills (not an issue in the western world)

Protect your life;control your eating,blaming the food industry will not help,they have been the usual suspects for decades,they are used to being labelled as the bad guys, for them it is one of the costs of operating in the extremely profitable food sector. For decades, they have never stopped increasing their bottom line and pleasing their stockholders. Meanwhile their customers are consuming too much of their products and an increasing large number of them have been developing diet related illness.
The food industry has been laughing all the way to the bank,whilst being sued,derided,blamed.
No one has ever gone broke from selling fast food.

All this time people are getting fatter and incurring diet related illnesses. Along the way the food industry has developed a thick skin in order to protect their business, for instance a fizzy soft drink is comprised mainly of water and cheap flavourings sold for a massive mark up. And there is no legislation or recommendations on how much you should drink unlike alcohol. In the long term which is more dangerous alcohol or fizzy drinks? they can both impair health and cause illness. Alcohol has a well known reputation,you know that

the more you drink,the increased likelihood that you will run into difficulties,either immediately or down the line.
On the other hand,if you over indulge in soft drinks, the effects are not immediately obvious, down a 500ml bottle of a sugary fizzy soft drink on a daily basis and a couple of years down the line,a diet related illness is likely to come your way.

The only thing the food industry fears is legislation. Legislation is the only thing that will work as it will cover the whole industry, multinationals like Pepsi and Coca cola will always bow to bad publicity,and try to make their products attuned to public opinion. But what about the small producers who are more driven by profit than bad publicity. If the big companies are shamed into not producing fatcrap,there are millions of small companies eager to take their place. Only legislation will stop this from happening.

The Final word

The words of Benjamin Franklin; "to lengthen thy life,lessen thy meals"

The only way to lose weight and to keep it off permanently,is to teach yourself to consume less calories on a daily basis,live an active lifestyle,in short you have to buy less to eat less.
If for example you were used to eating a takeaway chicken biriyani,accompanied with vegetable curry and peshwari nan by yourself, from now,that must be a meal for two or stretch to 2 meals. Get used to it. Just do it.

You can change everything,you hate about your life.

Good luck.
Nuff Said.

More from Perseverance Works.

Eat yourself to death by Culina Salus order from Amazon.com

You know deep inside your heart that the junk you are eating is ruining your health. That thought flashes in your mind every time, you go shopping for clothes, for food, every time you look in the mirror or stand on the scales, every time you eat another chocolate bar, or order that extra large pizza or order your fourth takeaway meal of the week. You know that you are killing yourself slowly, bite by bite, munch by munch, burger-by-burger, cake-by-cake, fizzy drink by fizzy drink. You are slowly eating yourself to death and to be honest,you might be slightly concerned but you don't give a fuck.

The Winners Creed by Solicitus Civis Available to order from lulu.com

The winners creed on how to succeed after screwing up
This book is written for those of us, who have failed, messed up, screwed up, fallen and run from the field of battle, but on serious reflection have decided to get up ,dust ourselves off and enter the fray again. The Winners creed is the mindset you will need to adopt in order to succeed.
This book does not claim to have all the answers but is just trying to make you change your thinking and alter your mindset, because by changing the way you think, you will consequently change your life.
Now is time for you to change your life, it is up to you to take control of your destiny, as it has been said if anything is going to be, it is up to you.
It is time for you to decide that no matter what the politician's do, what the economy does, you must decide your own destiny, so when you are on your death bed, old and grey, the only tune you should be singing is Frank Sinatra's "My way".

Kitchen
Safety
Record
Created by Culina Salus

Kitchen daily diary refill sheets are no longer sent out by the Food Standards Agency.

Don't waste money photocopying or using up expensive printer ink or looking unprofessional with pieces of paper. Get the replacement now:

Kitchen Safety Record Created by Culina Salus

Contains:

- ➢ Daily dairy sheets
- ➢ Temperature records
- ➢ Contacts list
- ➢ Cleaning schedule
- ➢ Staff training record
- ➢ Supplier list

The daily diary sheet also incorporates the fridge temperature records, so you only need to record all information on one sheet.

Recommended for **ALL** kitchens including Hotels, Restaurants, Schools, Colleges, Hospitals, Nursing homes, Takeaways, Cafes, Mobile catering vans, Home caterers, Church and Community halls-*wherever food is prepared for members of the public.*

- ➢ *Order now at* Amazon.co.uk *by entering:* kitchen safety record *or* culina salus *into the search box.*

Culina Salus,a veteran of the catering industry with decades of extensive experience as a chef,chef and catering manager, event caterer ,food safety trainer working for companies such as Hilton Hotel,The BBC, Camberwell college of Arts,Tropical dream village in Malindi Kenya, Scolarest and Compass catering

- ➢ **Abide by Food Safety Regulations, keep safe and legally compliant,get your copy now at Amazon.co.uk by entering:** kitchen safety record **or** culina salus **into the search box.**

Safe food depends on a hygienic and well managed kitchen

Available to order from Amazon.co.uk